Anti-IgE Therapy in Asthma and Allergy

Anti-IgE Therapy in Asthma and Allergy

Syed Hasan Arshad, DM, MRCP

Director of the David Hide Asthma and Allergy Centre, Isle of Wight, UK and Director of Clinical Trials, Department of Medical Specialties, Southampton General Hospital, Southampton, UK

K Suresh Babu, MD, DNB

Clinical Research Fellow, Respiratory, Cell and Molecular Biology Research Division, University of Southampton School of Medicine, Southampton, UK

Stephen T Holgate, BSc, MD, DSc, FRCP, FRCPath, FIBiol, CBiol, FmedSci

Medical Research Council Professor of Immunopharmacology at the University of Southampton, Southampton General Hospital, Southampton, UK

MARTIN DUNITZ

© 2001 Martin Dunitz Ltd, a member of
the Taylor & Francis group

First published in the United Kingdom in 2001 by
Martin Dunitz Ltd
The Livery House
7–9 Pratt Street
London NW1 0AE

Tel: +44 (0) 207 482 2202
Fax: +44 (0) 207 267 0159
E-mail: info.dunitz@tandf.co.uk
Website: http://www.dunitz.co.uk

A CIP record for this book is
available from the British Library.

ISBN 1 84184 0904

Printed and bound in Italy by Printer Trento S.r.l.

Cover image: Interactions between CD4 T cells and B cells
that are important in IgE synthesis. Adapted with permission
from Busse WW, Lemanske RF. Advances in immunology: asthma.
NJEM 2001;**344**:353. Copyright © 2001
Massachusetts Medical Society. All rights reserved.

Contents

Preface

The discovery by Prausnitz and Küstner in 1921 of reagin, the circulating substance that could passively transfer the immediate allergic response from one individual to another, stimulated a 50-year search for the molecular basis of this phenomenon. The identification of reagin as IgE independently by Ishizakas and Johansson in the late 1960s provided the rational basis for diseases such as rhinitis, asthma and food allergy and a legitimate target for novel therapeutics. Almost 25 years were to pass before it was clearly shown that a monoclonal antibody directed against that part of the IgE molecule that is encrypted by the high- and low-affinity IgE receptors on effector cells could dramatically remove circulating and tissue IgE by forming small complexes that are easily cleared without cross-linking IgE on the surface of effector cells and, therefore, failing to produce anaphylactic responses. The fully humanized monoclonal antibody omalizumab (Xolair™) has these properties. It has been clearly demonstrated that when administered at 2–4 weekly intervals this therapy has markedly beneficial effects on multiple outcome measures in allergic asthma.

This pocketbook provides an illustrative summary of the role of IgE in asthma and allied allergic disorders and the effects of anti-IgE treatment. With little new having been introduced into the armamentarium for asthma therapy in the last three decades other than improvements in β_2-adrenoceptor agonists, corticosteroids and cysteinyl leukotriene antagonists, the introduction of omalizumab is likely to provide a new way of treating allergic disorders with effects that extend beyond a single affected organ and tissue. Its precise role in treatment guidelines will need to be carefully evaluated, but its clear efficacy and safety provide a clear statement about the importance of IgE across the full spectrum of allergic disease.

Syed Hasan Arshad
K Suresh Babu
Stephen T Holgate
March 2001

What is asthma and allergy?

What is asthma?

Asthma is a chronic inflammatory disease of the airways and manifests clinically as intermittent cough and wheezing in response to exposure to allergenic and non-allergenic stimuli. The severity of asthma varies widely among individuals. In most patients the symptoms are mild and intermittent. However, in some patients it is a life-threatening disease which severely affects their quality of life.

The National Heart, Lung, and Blood Institute (NHLBI)/World Health Organization (WHO) expert panel report defines asthma as (Figure 1):

> a chronic inflammatory disorder of the airways in which many cells and cellular elements play a role, in particular, mast cells, eosinophils, T lymphocytes, neutrophils, and epithelial cells. In susceptible individuals, this inflammation causes recurrent episodes of wheezing, breathlessness, chest tightness, and cough, particularly at night and/or in the early morning. These symptoms are usually associated with widespread but variable airflow limitation that is at least partly reversible either spontaneously or with treatment. The inflammation also causes an associated increase in airway responsiveness to a variety of stimuli.

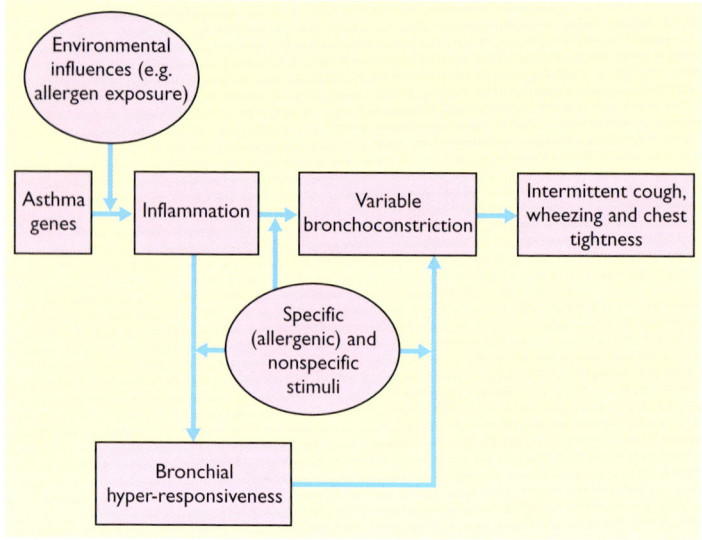

Figure 1 *Development of allergic inflammation in asthma and relationship to bronchial hyper-responsiveness and symptoms.*

Pathophysiology of asthma

Clinical features

Episodic cough and wheeze with chest tightness and difficulty in breathing are characteristic symptoms. These symptoms are usually most marked in the morning or at night. The cough is usually dry but may be productive of mucoid sputum. In some patients, cough is the only symptom. Most mild-to-moderate asthmatics wheeze on exposure to exogenous triggers, but in severe asthma, persistent wheezing may occur.

In mild asthma, physical examination may be entirely normal. However, in more severe forms, breathlessness may be apparent and chest auscultation may reveal inspiratory and/or expiratory wheezing. During an exacerbation the patient is breathless, apprehensive and restless. Tachycardia and tachypnoea is almost always present, and speech may be difficult. Wheezing may be heard without stethoscope, but in most severe forms the chest may be silent.

On lung function tests, a typical obstructive-type defect is often noted with a prominent reduction in forced vital capacity in one second (FEV$_1$). The variable bronchoconstriction can be demonstrated from diurnal and day-to-day variability in the peak expiratory flow rates (Figure 2).

Pathology

The clinical features of asthma are due to the airway narrowing causing obstruction to airflow. This narrowing results from the underlying inflammation, and has three elements:

■ Excessive bronchial smooth muscle contraction
■ Thickening of bronchial wall
■ Excessive secretions in the lumen

Excessive bronchial smooth muscle contraction
Inflammatory mediators such as histamine, bradykinin, prostaglandins and leukotrienes act directly on their specific

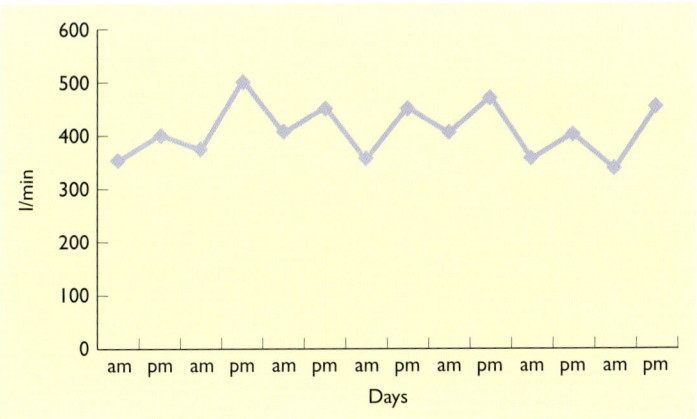

Figure 2 *Diurnal and day-to-day variability in peak flow is characteristic of asthma.*

receptors to cause bronchoconstriction. Stimulation of the cholinergic receptors causes bronchoconstriction, whereas adrenaline acting on the β_2-receptors has the opposite effect. The physiological role of non-adrenergic, non-cholinergic nerves is unclear.

In asthma, the smooth muscles contract easily and excessively following exposure to inflammatory mediators, perhaps due to the heightened sensitivity of their receptors. This feature is called bronchial hyper-responsiveness and can be demonstrated in the laboratory by inhalation of stimuli such as histamine or metha-choline.

Thickening of the bronchial wall
Thickening of the bronchial wall is due to inflammatory and fibrotic changes. Increased microvascular permeability allows plasma exudation into the mucosa, causing oedema, and cellular infiltration of eosinophils, mast cells and mononuclear cells. This causes swelling of the airway wall and loss of elastic recoil pressure, contributing to airway narrowing and hyper-responsiveness.

As the epithelium is damaged, the myofibroblasts lying beneath the epithelium proliferate and lay down collagen, causing thickening of the basement membrane (Figure 3). Other changes include hypertrophy and hyperplasia of airway smooth muscle, increase in goblet cell numbers and remodelling of the airway connective tissue. These changes may lead to irreversible obstruction in chronic asthma.

Excessive secretions in the lumen
Bronchial biopsy in asthmatic patients shows that the epithelium is fragile, and damaged epithelial cells are found in the sputum. Increased mucous secretion, with exuded protein and cell debris, comprises the mucous plug. Impaired ciliary function encourages retention of thick mucus in the lumen. During severe exacerbation, the lumen of the airway is blocked by thick mucus, plasma proteins and cell debris (Figure 4).

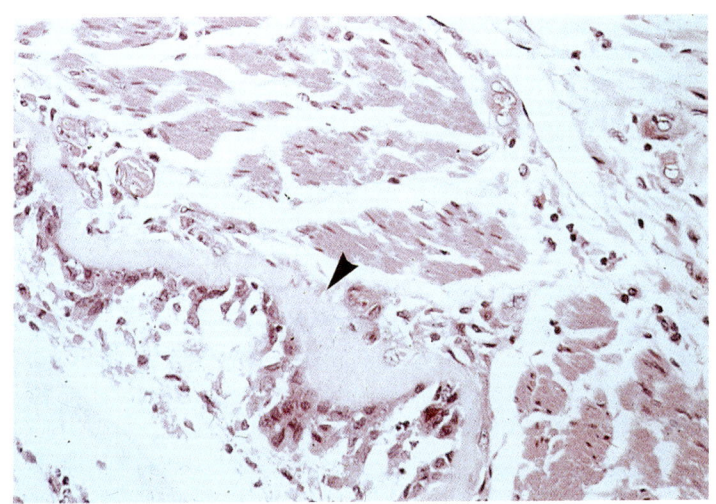

Figure 3 *Thickening of the basement membrane with deposition of collagen may lead to irreversible obstruction in chronic asthma.*

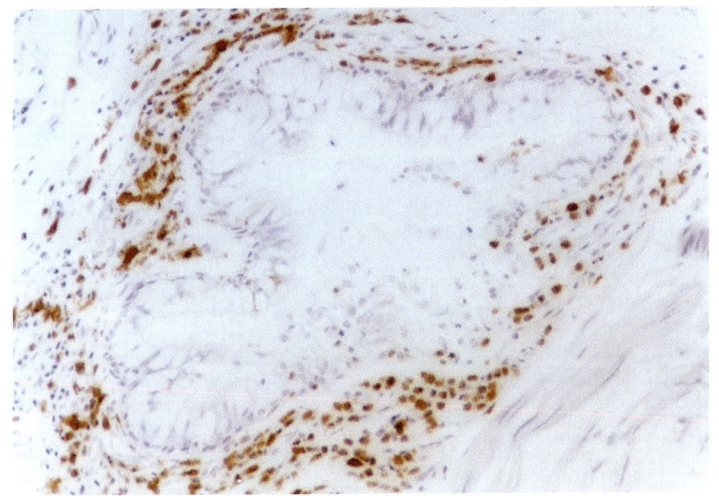

Figure 4 *Cross-section through airways showing mucosal oedema and mucous plugging. During severe exacerbation, the lumen of the airway is blocked by thick mucus, plasma proteins and cell debris.*

What is allergy?

Allergy is defined as an inappropriate or harmful immune response to foreign substances that are otherwise not harmful to the body. These substances are called allergens, and the immune response is mediated largely, though not exclusively, by the antibody IgE. Common sources of allergens include house dust mites, airborne pollens of grass, trees and weeds, domestic pets, mould spores and foods. IgE-mediated allergic disorders include allergic asthma, allergic rhinoconjunctivitis, atopic dermatitis, and some forms of occupational, food, drug and insect venom allergy. Atopy, the genetic propensity to produce IgE, is a prerequisite for the development of these disorders, and can usually be confirmed by positive responses on skin prick test (or the presence of specific IgE in the serum) to common allergens.

Allergens are introduced into the body through respiratory, gastrointestinal or conjunctival mucosa, with the exception of insect stings or drug allergies, where they may be injected through the skin. Initial exposure causes sensitization and production of IgE antibodies, specific to the allergen. Subsequent exposures may lead to immune reaction and disease. Clinical manifestations of this reaction depend on the organ involved. For example, in the airways this reaction causes asthma, whereas in the nasal and conjunctival mucosa, it may cause rhinoconjunctivitis.

Epidemiology of asthma and allergy

Natural history

Sensitization to food allergens, such as cows' milk and eggs is common in early childhood, and is associated with a high prevalence of eczema and food allergic reactions. By the age of 4 years, the majority of children tolerate food allergens, but many of these children develop allergies to inhalant allergens such as house dust mite and pollen, with a concomitant increase in the prevalence of asthma and hay fever in later childhood. This is termed 'allergy march'. Nearly 50% of children and adolescents 'grow out' of asthma and rhinitis as they approach adulthood. However, young adults may develop asthma or rhinitis for the first time. A family history of similar disorders is a common denominator in these individuals.

Prevalence of allergy

Prevalence of atopy, as defined by the presence of positive skin test or specific IgE to one or more allergens, ranges from 30% to 50% in various studies. However, not all atopic individuals develop allergic disease. More than a quarter of the population develop one or more allergic disorders (Figure 5). These range from mild hay fever to life-threatening asthma or systemic anaphylaxis. The International Study of Asthma and Allergy in Childhood (ISAAC), using standardized questionnaires, obtained comparable

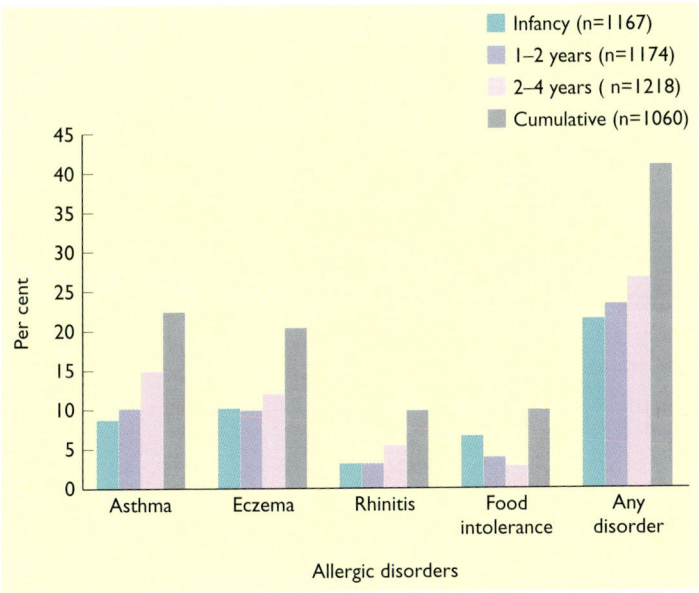

Figure 5 *Prevalence of allergic disorders in early childhood. Data from a whole population birth cohort study. Reproduced with permission from Tariq et al (1997).*

information on the prevalence of asthma and allergy from different parts of the world. This confirmed a high prevalence of these disorders in most developed countries. Serial studies in the same population have confirmed a rise in the prevalence of asthma and other allergic disorders during the last few decades.

Asthma

In the ISAAC study, the prevalence of self-reported ever asthma in children in the industrialized world was around 20–30%. Using more stringent criteria of current wheezing and bronchial hyper-responsiveness, the prevalence of asthma varies between 8% and 15%. An estimated 17.8 million people suffer from this disease in the USA alone. The direct cost of asthma in the USA was estimated to be around $11 billion. Indirect cost is more difficult to estimate accurately, but this is substantial in terms of lost productivity and school days. The cost is enormous, though 80% of the resources are consumed by 20% of the asthmatic population, who have more severe disease.

Allergic rhinitis

The prevalence of seasonal allergic rhinitis (hay fever) is said to be around 10–12%, and a similar figure is quoted for perennial allergic rhinitis. As with asthma, the prevalence of allergic rhinitis is increasing. The cost of allergic rhinitis is high, primarily because of the high prevalence of this disease. It was estimated to be in excess of $3 billion in the USA in 1996. Indirect cost of loss of work productivity and reduced performance and learning, is additional.

Atopic eczema

The prevalence rates of atopic eczema in early childhood range from 10%–12%. In the vast majority, atopic eczema improves, although in nearly 50% some eczema lesions persist into adulthood. Moderate to severe atopic eczema has a major impact on the quality of life of children and their parents.

Food allergy

Food allergy is defined as adverse reactions to food with an immunological basis. Cows' milk, eggs, fruits, nuts, fish and wheat are the commonest food allergens. Common symptoms of food allergy include urticaria/angioedema, vomiting, diarrhoea, and, rarely, anaphylactic shock. Allergy to cows' milk (3–4%) and eggs (2–3%) is common in infancy but rarely persists beyond 3 years of age. Peanut allergy affects around 0.5% of the population of all ages.

Anaphylaxis

Less than 0.1% of the unselected population report ever having an anaphylactic episode in their life. Common causes of anaphylaxis include drugs, insect venom, latex and foods, especially nuts. However, patients with severe food, drug or latex allergy live in constant fear of an inadvertent exposure and subsequent, potentially life-threatening, reaction.

2

What is immunoglobulin E?

History of allergy

Allergic disorders have been described as far back as 3000 BC, when King Menes, who ruled Egypt, was killed by a hornet. Greek scholars described the clinical symptoms of asthma, although this encompassed different types of breathing problem. In 1552, Dr Carden, a contemporary Italian physician, cured the Archbishop of St Andrew's from asthma by getting rid of the feather quilt and pillows which he had used. In 1586, Marcello Donati of Germany described an aristocrat whose lips swelled whenever he indulged in eggs.

The first skin prick test under medical auspices seems to have been carried out by Pierre Borel in 1656. During the 17th century, German authors described weakness, fainting and asthma in certain subjects exposed to cats, mice, dogs and horses. Dr Bostock, who had symptoms of his eyes and chest, described hay fever, but the classic experiments of Charles Blackley, in 1873, provided the proof that hay fever was caused by grass pollen.

In 1839 the French physiologist Magendie described anaphylactic shock and death in dogs repeatedly injected with foreign proteins. Von Behring coined the term hypersensitivity to describe the exaggerated response and even death following a second dose of diphtheria toxin in animals. Portier and Richet first used the term anaphylaxis in 1902, when they described a clinical shock syndrome encountered in dogs given otherwise innocuous doses of toxin after a previous experience with the same substance. The term allergy, meaning 'changed reactivity', was originally defined by Clemens von Priquet in 1906 as an altered capacity of the body to react to foreign substances. In the subsequent years, the mechanisms of anaphylactic reaction were further expanded by the experiments of Shultz and Dale on intestinal and uterine smooth muscles. Cellular involvement in the process of anaphylaxis was proposed; it was stated that the small amounts of antibody required were in fact affixed to the surface of appropriate target cells, and any subsequent interaction would result in cell damage and a consequent shock-like syndrome.

History of IgE

Allergy is often equated with the type I hypersensitivity reaction – an immediate hypersensitivity reaction mediated by IgE. This relationship between serum IgE and allergic diseases was recognized in the early 1900s when Otto Carl W. Prausnitz (1876–1963) and his colleague Heinz Küstner (1897–1963) identified 'reagin'. They took serum from Küstner, who was allergic to fish, and injected it into the skin of Prausnitz. When the fish antigen was subsequently injected into the sensitized site, there was an immediate wheal and flare reaction. This reaction, called the P-K reaction, was the basis for the earliest bioassay for IgE activity.

It was not until 1966 that Kimishige and Teruko Ishizaka identified the reaginic antibody. They obtained serum from an allergic individual and immunized rabbits with it to prepare anti-isotype antiserum. The rabbit antiserum was then allowed to react with each class of human antibody known at that time (i.e. IgG, IgA, IgM and IgD). In this way, each of the known anti-isotype antibodies was precipitated and removed from the rabbit antiserum. The one that remained was an anti-isotype antibody specific for an unidentified class of antibody. This anti-isotype antibody turned out to completely block the P-K reaction. This was called gamma E (erythema) globulin – immunoglobulin E. In 1968, the WHO international conference concluded that this new class of immunoglobulin, IgE, was the true mediator of the biological and immunological features formerly ascribed to reaginic antibodies.

Immunoglobulin E

Like other antibodies, IgE comprises two identical light (L) chains and two identical heavy (H) chains, each chain being made up of 110 amino acids; the chains are called immunoglobulin domains, and are covalently linked by disulphide bonds (Figure 6). The L chain has one N-terminal variable (V_L) domain and one constant

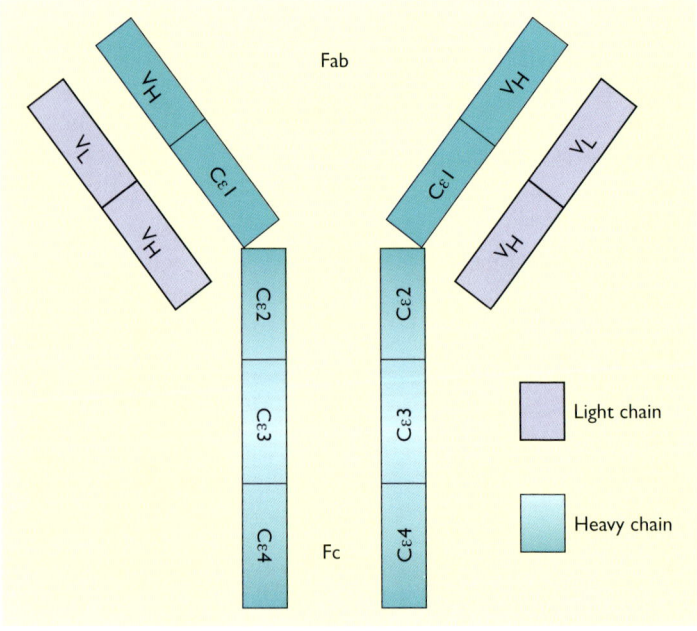

Figure 6 *The domain structure of IgE.*

(C_L) domain. Likewise, the H chain consists of one N-terminal V (V_H) domain and four C (C_H) domains. The antibody class is determined by the C_H sequence designated as Cε for IgE. A given B-cell produces an antibody with one specificity as defined by the V_L and V_H combination, but during an antibody response, it can 'switch' classes.

The ε heavy chain is similar to the μ chain of IgM, in that it has four constant region domains (Cε1–Cε4). Cε2 takes the hinge region in IgE, and papain digestion cleaves between Cε1 and Cε2 to produce the Fab fragment and the Fc fragment that contains Cε2–Cε4. The antigen-binding site is present in the Fab fragment, while the Fc portion is the crystallizable fragment. There are two antigen-binding sites in IgE, which are formed by the pairing of V_L and V_H domains, while the cell-receptor combining sites are formed by the dimerization of the ε chains. Studies with recombination peptides and chimeric antibodies have mapped the receptor-binding site to the Cε3 domain of IgE.

IgE has a molecular weight of 190 000 and has a very low serum concentration (0.3 μg/l). The half-life of free IgE in the serum is about 2–3 days, but once IgE is bound to its receptors on mast cells and basophils, it is stable in the bound state for a number of weeks.

Receptors for IgE

The activity of IgE depends on its ability to bind to specific receptors for the Fc portion of the ε heavy chain. Two classes of Fcε receptors have been identified, designated as FcεRI and FcεRII (or CD23).

High-affinity receptor (FcεRI)
The high-affinity receptor is predominantly expressed on mast cells, basophils and antigen-presenting cells (APCs) and not on

their precursors in the circulation. The high affinity of this receptor ($K_D = 1–2 \times 10^{-9}$ M) enables it to bind to IgE despite its low serum concentrations. The FcεRI receptor has four polypeptide chains: an α-chain and a β-chain and two identical disulphide-linked γ-chains. FcεRI interacts with the C_H3/C_H3 and C_H4/C_H4 domains of the IgE molecule via the two immunoglobulin-like domains of the α-chain (Figure 7). FcεRI either wraps around a single Cε3 domain to make contact with both sides, or interacts with opposite faces of the Cε3 domains on one side of IgE. The β-chain spans the plasma membrane four times, and the two γ-chains extend a considerable distance into the cytoplasm. Allergen-mediated cross-linkage of the bound IgE results in

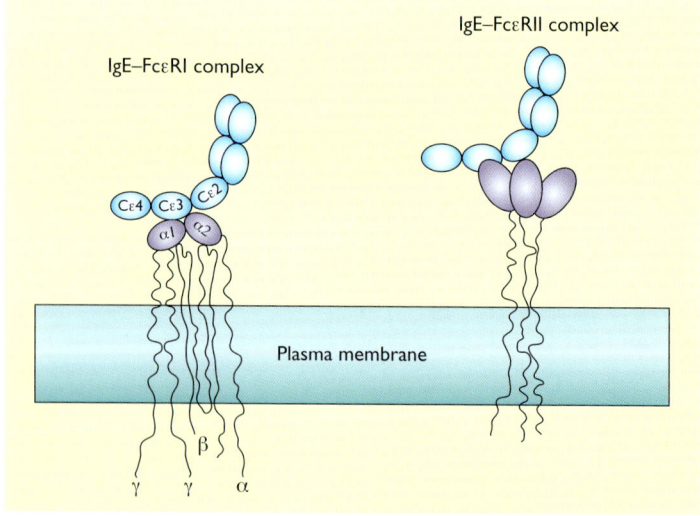

Figure 7 *The IgE–FcεRI receptor complex has a 1 : 1 stoichiometry with the binding sites in Cε3 and Cα2. The IgE–FcεRII complex has an extracellular C-terminus and an N-terminal cytoplasmic sequence.*

aggregation of the FcεRI receptors and rapid tyrosine phosphorylation, which initiates the process of mast cell degranulation.

Low-affinity receptor (FcεRII or CD23)

FcεRII is the low-affinity IgE receptor, with a K_D of 1×10^{-6} M and is specific for the C_H3/C_H3 domain of IgE. It belongs to the family of C-type lectins. CD23 is a 45-kDa polypeptide chain with extracellular structural motifs, a transmembrane sequence and a cytoplasmic tail. The cytoplasmic tail can be either of two types: CD23a or CD23b. Allergen cross-linkage of IgE bound to the FcεRII receptors results in activation of B-cells, eosinophils and alveolar macrophages, and blockade of this receptor with a monoclonal antibody leads to diminished IgE secretion by the B-cells. Interestingly, CD23 appears to act in both the upregulation and downregulation of IgE synthesis, and atopic individuals have higher levels of CD23 on their lymphocytes and macrophages. CD23–IgE interaction provides an important mechanism whereby allergen-specific IgE can augment cellular and humoral immune responses in settings of recurrent allergen exposure.

The events underlying mast cell and basophil degranulation have many features in common. Mast cell degranulation is predominantly initiated by allergen cross-linkage of bound IgE, although other stimuli can also initiate this process. Allergen cross-links the bound IgE (fixed IgE) to the high-affinity FcεRI receptor on a mast cell or a basophil, leading to degranulation of these cells and release of mediators of inflammation. The primary mediators released are histamine, proteases, eosinophil and neutrophil chemotactic factor and heparin, clinically manifesting as the immediate reaction (Figure 8). The secondary mediators include platelet-activating factor, cytokines, leukotrienes, prostaglandins and bradykinin, and these cause the late-phase reactions.

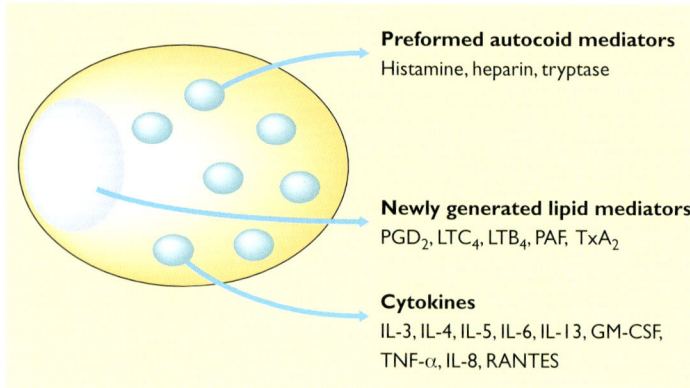

Figure 8 *IgE-mediated mast cell degranulation leads to release of mediators, which are essentially chemoattractants (IL-5, IL-8, TNF-α, LTB$_4$, PAF), inflammatory activators (histamine, PAF, tryptase and kinins) and spasmogens (histamine, PGD$_2$, LTC$_4$ and LTD$_4$). LT, leukotriene; PAF, platelet-activating factor; TxA$_2$, thromboxane A$_2$; IL, interleukin; PGD$_2$, prostaglandin D$_2$; GM-CSF, granulocyte–monocyte colony-stimulating factor.*

The release of these mediators in the different organ systems leads to varying manifestations (Figure 9). Intravenous administration of allergen leads to anaphylactic shock, while asthma and allergic rhinitis is apparent when the allergen encounters the airway mucosa. Asthma, allergic rhinitis and atopic dermatitis are almost invariably associated with elevated IgE levels. It is believed that allergen-specific IgE is generally connected with the induction of allergic airway symptoms. In the airway mucosa, these mediators of immediate hypersensitivity reactions rapidly induce mucosal oedema, increased mucous production and smooth muscle constriction, eventually leading to an inflammatory infiltration.

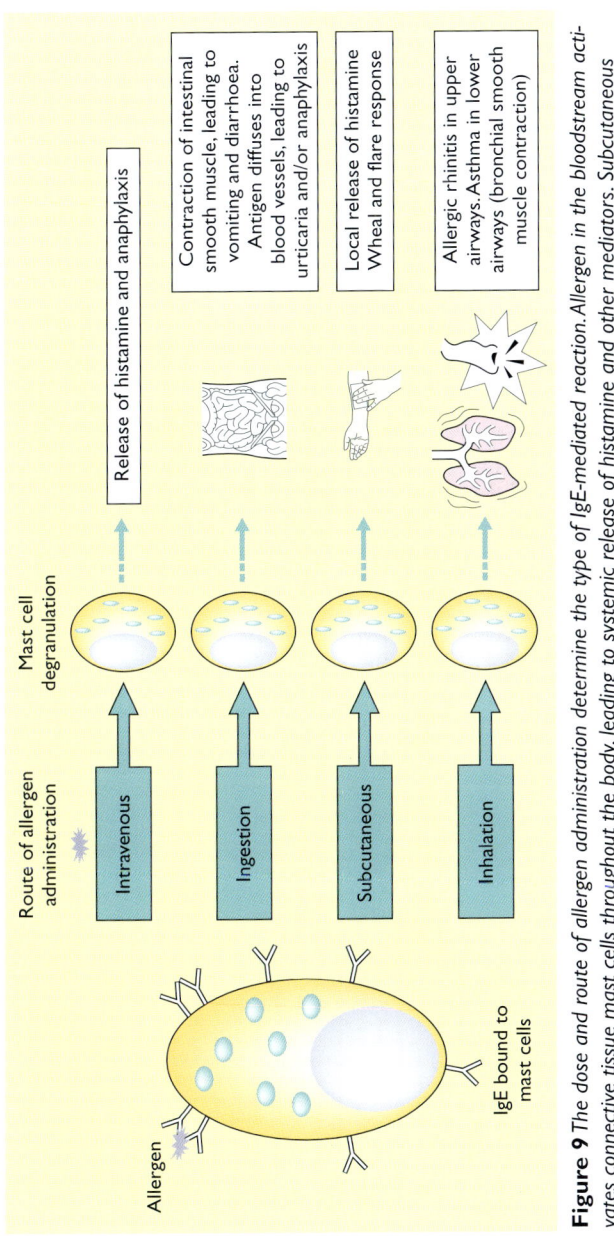

Figure 9 The dose and route of allergen administration determine the type of IgE-mediated reaction. Allergen in the bloodstream activates connective tissue mast cells throughout the body, leading to systemic release of histamine and other mediators. Subcutaneous administration causes a local inflammatory reaction. Inhaled allergen activates mucosal mast cells, leading to bronchoconstriction and increased mucous secretion. Ingested allergen causes vomiting due to intestinal smooth muscle contraction and diarrhoea due to increased intestinal secretion.

17

3 Synthesis and regulation of IgE

Serum IgE levels correlate well with allergic airway disease, and genetic analyses of families have shown bronchial hyper-responsiveness to be linked to serum IgE levels. IgE is set apart from other immunoglobulins by its very low plasma levels, and even in severe disease, where IgE levels are in excess of 100 times normal, values rarely approach baseline levels of other immunoglobulins. Thus, the levels of IgE are tightly controlled to prevent the potentially lethal effects of IgE-dependent inflammation.

Regulation of IgE response

Role of helper T-cells

Adaptive immune responses are broadly categorized into two antagonistic subtypes – Th_1 and Th_2 – each with its own set of cytokine profiles. Th_1 cells produce interleukin (IL)-2, interferon (IFN)-γ and TNF-β, whereas Th_2 cells produce IL-4, IL-5, IL-6, IL-10 and IL-13. The cytokine products of Th_1 and Th_2 cells are mutually inhibitory for the differentiation and effector functions of the reciprocal phenotypes. The functions of Th_1 and Th_2 cells correlate with their distinct cytokines. Th_1 cytokines activate cytotoxic and inflammatory functions and are involved in cell-mediated immune reactions, whereas Th_2 cytokines encourage antibody production, particularly IgE responses. The type 2 cytokine IL-4 is crucial for the production of IgE in B-cells, whereas the level of co-production of the type 1 cytokine IFN-γ determines the immunoglobulin isotype.

Role of genetic factors

The genetic constitution of an individual determines the level of IgE response induced by an antigen. The genetic component is apparent from family studies, where, if both parents are allergic, the chance that a child will be allergic is 50%, while when only one parent is allergic, the chance that a child will manifest a type I response is 30%. The human major histocompatibility complex (MHC) includes genes coding for HLA class II molecules, which are involved in the recognition and presentation of exogenous peptides. Allergenic peptides with low or high affinity for MHC molecules would confer relatively weak or strong signals, facilitating deviation towards a Th_2 cell phenotype and thereby allergy. There is also accruing evidence that a low T-cell receptor α/δ region modulates IgE responses. The close correlation between the total and specific IgE makes it difficult to determine whether the locus controls specific IgE reactions to a particular antigen or confers generalized IgE responsiveness. Nevertheless, linkage was strongest with highly purified antigens, suggesting that this locus primarily influences specific responses.

Role of antigen

Antigen dose, the mode of presentation and sometimes the adjuvant affect the IgE response. The biochemical properties of the antigens significantly influence the direction of the immune response (Th_1 or Th_2). By definition, allergens including products of some infectious organisms give rise to a predominant Th_2 response and high serum IgE levels. Furthermore, many allergens are enzymatically active, and this protease selectively cleaves surface CD23 of B-cells, potentially interrupting a negative regulator of IgE production. IgE response also depends on the antigen dosing. Presenting an antigen transmucosally at a low dose effectively induces a Th_2-driven IgE response. The route of exposure to allergen can also influence the IgE response. Antigen administered through the respiratory tract is highly immunogenic, in contrast to antigen encountered through other routes.

Role of IL-4 and IL-13

IgE production requires at least two distinct signals (Figure 10). The first signal is provided by the cytokines IL-4 and IL-13. IL-4 is produced by T-cells, although mast cells, basophils and eosinophils may also produce IL-4, whereas IL-13 is produced in addition by the NK cells. IL-4 and IL-13 share the common α-chain of the IL-4 receptor (IL-4Rα). Engagement of this moiety with either ligand results in translocation to the nucleus of signal transducer and activator of transcription 6 (STAT-6), which stim-

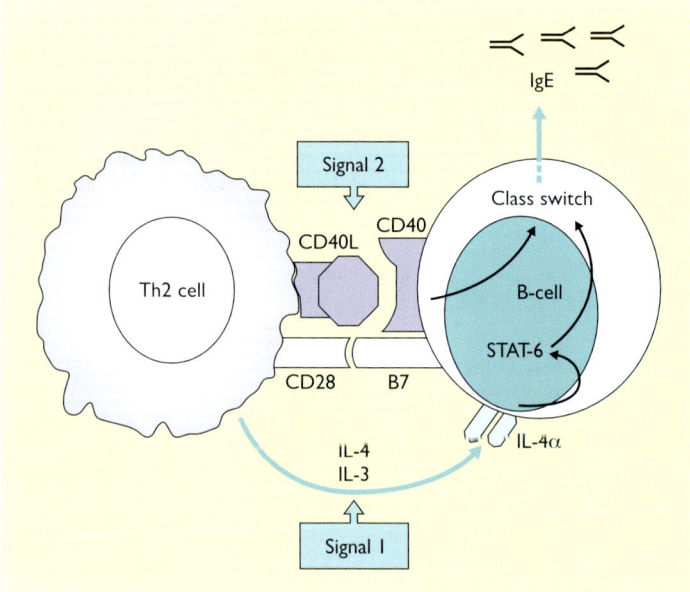

Figure 10 *Engagement of T-cell receptor by MHC class II molecules leads to expression of CD40 ligand (CD40L), which engages CD40. CD40L-induced aggregation of CD40b triggers the expression of B7 (CD80). Interaction of B7 with CD28 on the surface of T-cells delivers the costimulatory signals inducing secretion of IL-4. IL-4 binds to its receptor IL-4R (signal 1), which in conjunction with CD40 ligation (signal 2) triggers the IgE isotype switch, B-cell proliferation and expansion of IgE-producing cells.*

ulate transcription of the Cε gene locus containing the exons encoding the constant region domains of the IgE ε heavy chain.

The second signal is delivered by the interaction of CD40L on the surface of T-cells with CD40, a costimulatory molecule on the B-cell membrane. This activates a genetic rearrangement (deletional switch recombination) that brings into proximity all the elements of a functional ε heavy chain. The product is a complete multi-exon gene encoding the full ε heavy chain. The combination of these signals causes class switching to IgE and B-cell proliferation (Figure 11). Once initiated, the IgE response can be further amplified by basophils, mast cells and eosinophils, which can also drive IgE production (Figure 12).

There are other factors that play a role in the regulation of IgE levels. Cross-linking of FcεRI upregulates its own expression and enhances the ability of mast cells sensitized with IgE to degranulate in response to antigen challenge. However, CD23, the low-

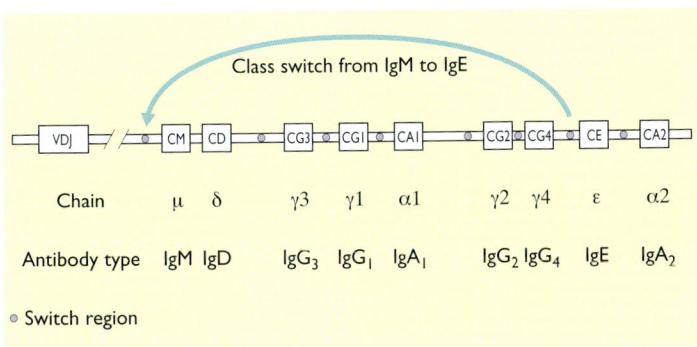

Figure 11 *The human immunoglobulin heavy chain locus. Initially, B-cells transcribe VDJ gene and μ heavy chain, which is spliced to produce mRNA for IgM. The direction of the switch is determined by lymphokines secreted by T-cells. IL-4 and IL-13 promote the class switch to IgE, while IFN-γ inhibits this. Under the influence of IL-4 and IL-13, class switching to IgE occurs that brings together the VDJ gene and the Cε region, allowing a looping out and deletion of the intervening C genes.*

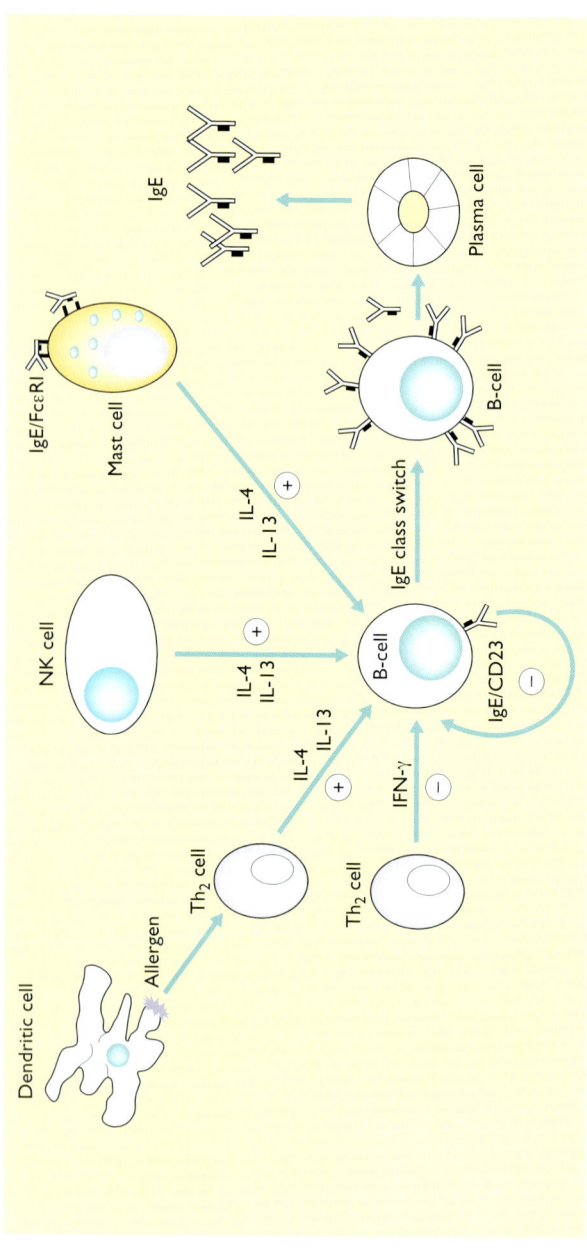

Figure 12 Th$_2$ cells provide signals for IgE production through IL-4 and IL-13. IgE secreted by plasma cells binds to FcεRI on mast cells and basophils. When the surface bound IgE is cross-linked by antigen, these cells express CD40L and secrete IL-4, which in turn stimulate IgE isotype switching, producing more IgE. NK cells also secrete IL-4 and IL-13 to promote IgE synthesis. In contrast, IFN-γ and IgE–CD23 interaction decrease IgE production.

affinity receptor, seems to serve principally as a negative regulator of IgE synthesis. Likewise, IFN-γ has a negative role in IgE synthesis by effectively inhibiting the class switching to IgE. In general, the nature of the antigen, the route of its entry and the genetic make-up of an individual tightly control IgE synthesis.

IgE-mediated degranulation

The consequences of IgE-mediated mast cell activation depend on the dose of antigen and the route of entry of the antigen. Only complexes having an IgE/allergen ratio of 2 : 1 or greater could induce degranulation.

The cytoplasmic domains of the high-affinity receptors are associated with protein tyrosine kinases. Cross-linking of FcϵRI receptors activates the tyrosine kinases, leading to the phosphorylation of the γ-subunit, β-subunit and phospholipase C. This phosphorylation activates a number of second messengers, resulting in an increase in membrane fluidity and the formation of calcium (Ca^{2+}) channels, leading to an influx of Ca^{2+} into the cell. The Ca^{2+} influx leads to the formation of arachidonic acid and also promotes the assembly of microtubules, which are necessary for the movement of the granules towards the plasma membrane. FcϵRI cross-linkage also activates membrane adenyl cyclase, leading to a transient increase in cAMP. The cAMP- dependent protein kinase phosphorylates the membrane proteins, resulting in swelling of the granules and release of the mediators. These inflammatory products elicit the familiar signs and symptoms of atopic diseases.

Allergic inflammation and the role of IgE

Allergic inflammation

A complex interplay of inflammatory cells and chemical mediators is responsible for allergic inflammation. First, exposure(s) to allergen leads to sensitization and production of IgE antibodies. During subsequent exposures, allergic reaction is initiated by IgE antibodies and orchestrated by T-lymphocytes, the major inflammatory cells being mast cells and eosinophils. Allergic inflammation has been extensively studied, in animal models and human subjects, with the events following experimental allergen challenge.

Sensitization

When antigen enters the body through the mucosal surfaces or skin, the antigen presenting cells such as macrophages, engulf the antigens. After processing, the antigen is presented to the naive T-helper cells (Th_0). This stimulates their differentiation (in the presence of IL-4) into Th_2-type lymphocytes, which in turn secrete a number of cytokines, including IL-4 and IL-13 (Figure 13). These cytokines cause proliferation and switching of B-cells (specific to the antigen) to IgE-producing B-cells and plasma cells. This IgE circulates in the blood and enters tissues, including airway mucosa and skin, where it is mostly bound to the high-affinity receptors (FcεRI) on the surface of mast cells, and low-affinity receptors (FcεRII) on eosinophils, macrophages and platelets. The attachment of IgE antibodies to specific receptors on mast cells

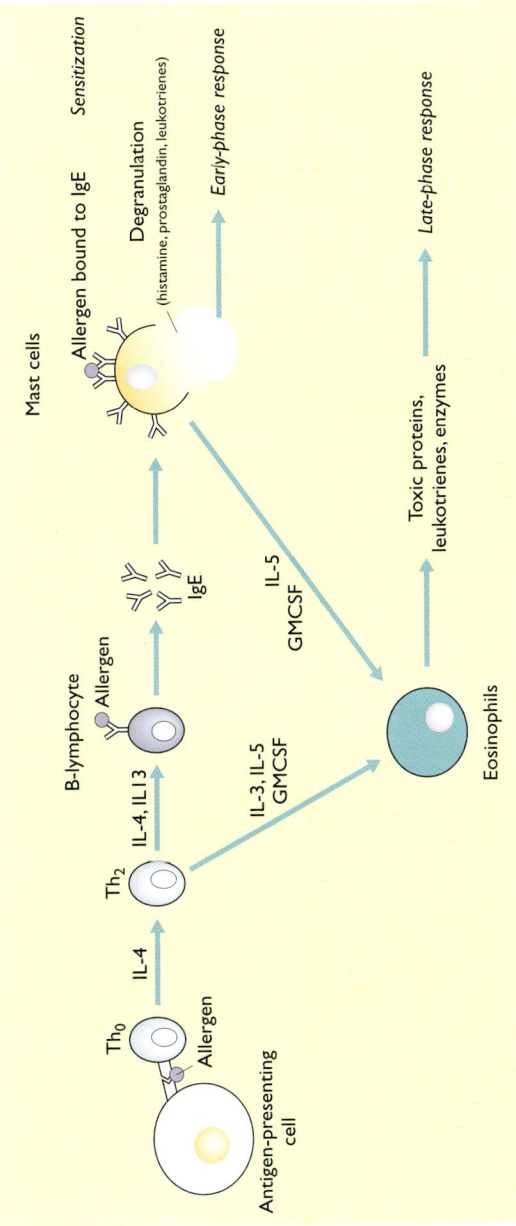

Figure 13 *Schematic representation of the mechanism of allergic inflammation.*

Antigen-presenting cell

Th₀ → Allergen

IL-4

Th₂

B-lymphocyte

IL-4, IL13

Allergen

IgE

IL-3, IL-5 GMCSF

Eosinophils

IL-5 GMCSF

Mast cells

Allergen bound to IgE

Degranulation (histamine, prostaglandin, leukotrienes)

Sensitization

Early-phase response

Toxic proteins, leukotrienes, enzymes

Late-phase response

sets the stage for an acute inflammatory response on subsequent antigen exposure.

Early-phase response

When an allergen penetrates the epithelium or skin of a sensitized individual, an early phase response is observed (Figure 14). This response is dependent on the cross-linking of Fab fragments of two adjacent IgE antibodies, on the surface of the mast cells, by allergen, resulting in the degranulation and release of preformed (histamine, heparin) and newly synthesized (prostaglandins, leukotrienes, platelet-activating factor and bradykinin) mediators. These mast cell-derived mediators enhance vascular dilatation, increased permeability of the venule and increased mucous secretion, resulting in oedema and congestion, typical of an acute-phase reaction. Histamine and

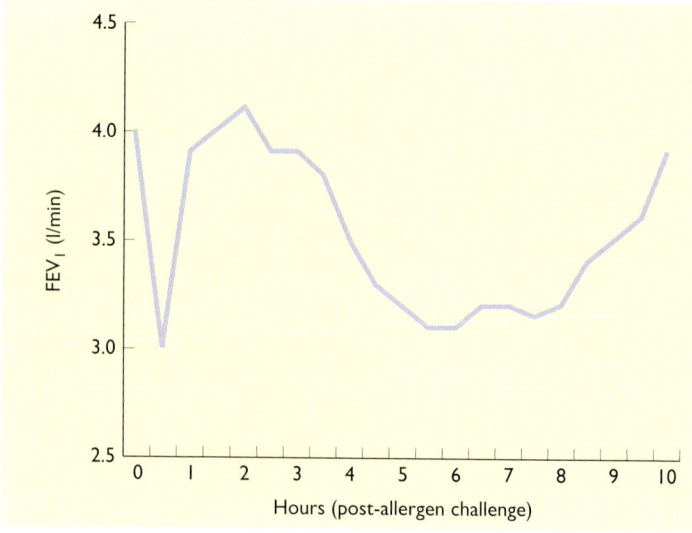

Figure 14 *Early and late asthmatic responses following allergen challenge. There is immediate bronchoconstriction (fall in FEV$_1$) soon after allergen inhalation, which improves over 2 h, to be followed by a prolonged decrease in FEV$_1$ over 4–10 h, post-challenge.*

leukotrienes are potent bronchoconstrictors. Histamine stimulates local type c neurones, leading to the release of several neuropeptides, including substance P, which further increase vascular permeability and cause stimulation of parasympathetic reflexes, augmenting mucous secretion and bronchoconstriction. These changes manifest clinically in cough and wheeze (lung), erythema, induration and itching (skin), sneezing and rhinorrhoea (nose) and itching and lacrimation (eyes).

Mast cells also release cytokines such as IL-3, IL-4, IL-5, granulocyte–macrophage colony-stimulating factor (GM-CSF) and TNF-α, which activate T- and B-lymphocytes, stimulate mast cells and attract eosinophils. IL-4 and TNF-α upregulate intercellular and vascular adhesion molecules, promoting stickiness of the endothelium to leukocytes and facilitating their passage into the tissues with the aid of TNF-α. This process takes a few hours to establish and results in the late-phase response.

Late-phase response

Clinically, the effect of the early-phase reaction diminishes after 30 min. This is followed by a relatively asymptomatic period, during which a plethora of cytokines and mediators, generated during the early phase, draw leukocytes to the tissues. IL-5, secreted from mast cells, lymphocytes and eosinophils, is the most important cytokine for eosinophils. Besides attracting them to the site of inflammation, it also causes their proliferation, activation and increased survival. Other eosinophilic cytokines are IL-3, GM-CSF and chemokines. Upon activation, eosinophils release mediators such as eosinophilic cationic protein (ECP), major basic protein (MBP), leukotrienes and prostaglandins. These and other mediators enhance inflammation and cause epithelial damage. Neutrophils, basophils and lymphocytes are also increased in numbers during the late phase.

The late-phase allergic response is observed 2–6 h later in a significant number (50–60%) of individuals with asthma and rhinitis, and manifests clinically with congestion, increased mucous production and bronchoconstriction. Airway responsiveness to specific and nonspecific stimuli is increased, possibly as a result of exposure of nerve endings to airway lumina following epithelial damage.

Chronic inflammation

With continued or repeated exposure to allergen, a state of chronic inflammation develops, with increased numbers of activated Th_2 cells, expressing mRNA for the secretion of IL-3, IL-4, IL-5 and GM-CSF. These cytokines are important in the continuation of inflammation and the attraction of mast cells and eosinophils. These cells cause further increases in histamine, prostaglandins and various cytokines. Similarly, activated eosinophils are found in the mucosa with a parallel increase in their toxic products, causing epithelial damage. Additional eosinophil products such as transforming growth factor-α and -β mediate local tissue repair and contribute to airway remodelling in chronic asthma. Increased permeability and cellular infiltration cause mucosal oedema. There is also glandular hyperplasia with increased secretion. Overall, the effects of continued cellular recruitment and release of mediators result in clinical symptoms of asthma and rhinitis. These processes may also account for the hyper-reactivity observed in the nose and airways.

Role of IgE

IgE is the major immunoglobulin isotype responsible for sensitization to allergen. This sensitization is a prerequisite for the development of IgE-mediated responses in these diseases. Evidence for and against the role of IgE in allergen-induced inflammation is summarized.

Evidence for the role of IgE

The development of asthma is linked to high levels of serum IgE, through a genetic defect present on chromosome 5. IgE plays a crucial role in the allergic immune responses. Most of the cells implicated in allergic responses bear IgE receptors and can be activated by cross-linking of the bound IgE, resulting in an early-phase response to allergen. The severity of the early-phase response is related to the degree of sensitivity to the allergen. IgE is also postulated to be involved in the late-phase response. The late asthmatic response in turn leads to airway inflammation and bronchial hyper-responsiveness to specific (allergen) and nonspecific (irritants) stimuli.

Atopy, as defined by positive skin prick test or the presence of specific IgE to common allergens, is associated with the development of asthma. Epidemiological evidence supporting the role of total IgE in asthma includes the correlation of elevated serum levels of IgE with self-reported asthma symptoms and airway hyper-responsiveness (Figure 15).

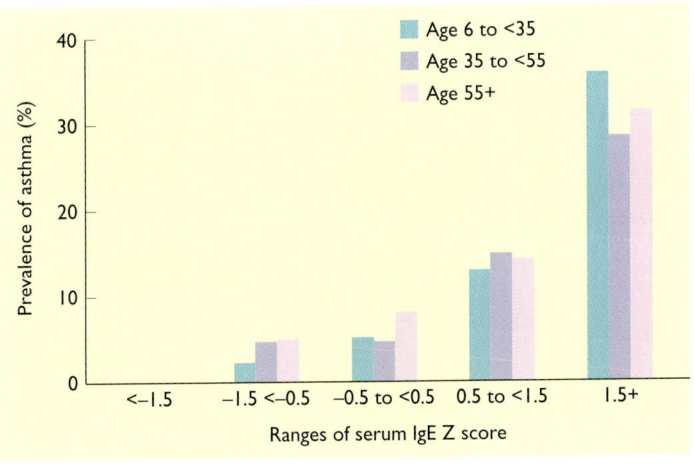

Figure 15 *In this population study, the prevalence of asthma was shown to be directly related to the level of IgE. Reproduced with permission from Burrows et al (1989). Copyright © 1989 Massachusetts Medical Society. All rights reserved.*

A high total serum IgE may not always be associated with atopy, as defined by positive skin prick test or the presence of specific IgE to common allergens. In vitro studies indicate that specific IgE determines allergen responsiveness but does not influence nonspecific bronchial responsiveness, which is more closely related to serum total IgE. Even non-atopic asthmatics manifest a higher level of total IgE compared to their non-atopic, non-asthmatic counterparts, and in these patients local IgE production can be demonstrated in airways. A recent report suggests that, in non-atopic individuals, asthma is more common if their serum total IgE is high.

Evidence against the role of IgE

Some investigators have not been able to find an association between total or specific IgE and the pattern of asthmatic responses following allergen inhalation, and suggest that the role of non-IgE (T-cell-directed) processes may be important, especially in the late asthmatic response. In a recent meta-analysis, it was suggested that less than 40% of the population attributable risk for asthma could be accounted for by atopy. Moreover, in the African population, serum levels of IgE were reported to be higher in non-asthmatics than in asthmatics.

Conclusion

The bulk of the evidence supports the suggestion that IgE plays an important signalling role in most patients with allergic disease. The recent availability of humanized monoclonal antibody against IgE has proven to be an invaluable tool to investigate the role of IgE in allergen-induced inflammation.

Current management of asthma and allergy

5

The management of allergic disorders includes allergen avoidance, specific allergen immunotherapy and pharmacotherapy. Allergen avoidance is indicated in all patients where there is evidence of clinical reactivity to a specific allergen. Although allergen avoidance should always be part of the overall management, this alone is rarely sufficient to control symptoms. Immunotherapy and pharmacotherapy can be used alone or in combination.

For some disorders such as food and latex allergy, avoidance is the only method currently available. In patients with allergic asthma, allergic rhinitis and atopic eczema, appropriate allergen avoidance may prevent exacerbations, and reduce symptoms and the need for medication. Non-allergenic triggers such as exposure to cigarette smoke should be identified and excluded from the patients' environment.

Most authorities agree that immunotherapy is effective in allergic rhinitis and insect venom allergy. The use of immunotherapy in asthma is less certain, and it is not effective in atopic dermatitis and food allergy. The treatment is expensive and requires frequent visits, and there is a potential for serious side-effects. For these reasons, immunotherapy is indicated only when allergen avoidance and pharmacotherapy have failed to suppress symptoms adequately.

Pharmacotherapy

Asthma

The growing awareness of the presence of inflammation even in mild asthma, and concerns regarding airway remodelling in untreated disease, have transformed asthma management during the past decade. Increased and early use of anti-inflammatory agents is now considered in all grades of asthma severity.

Pharmacotherapy is tailored to the grade of severity of the disease. The NHLBI/WHO expert panel report classifies asthma into four grades of severity: mild intermittent asthma, mild persistent asthma, moderate persistent asthma and severe persistent asthma (Table 1). By adhering to a management programme, an asthmatic should be able to achieve and maintain control of symptoms, prevent exacerbations, and maintain pulmonary function as close to normal levels as possible. Patients and parents of

Table 1 *Grades of asthma severity.*

	Grade 1 Mild intermittent	Grade 2 Mild persistent	Grade 3 Moderate	Grade 4 Severe
Day symptoms	< 1/week	>1/week	>1/day	Continuous
Nocturnal symptoms	< 2/month	> 2/month	>1/week	Most nights
FEV_1	Normal	Normal	>60% to 80% predicted	≤60%
Peak flow variability	<20%	20–30%	>30%	>30%
Bronchodilator requirement	Occasional	<1/day	Daily use	Several times/day
Exacerbation	Hours to days, may not require oral steroids	Affect activity, may require oral steroids	Affect activity and sleep, require oral steroids	Frequent and may be severe

Presence of one of the features of severity puts the patients in the higher grade (adapted from Global Strategy for Asthma Management and Prevention. NHLBI/WHO Workshop Report. NIH publication 1995; No. 95: 3659).

asthmatic children should be given information and education to enable them to take control of their disease.

Drugs used in the long-term treatment of asthma can be broadly classified into prophylactic and rescue medications. Prophylactic treatment is primarily with anti-inflammatory agents, and inhaled corticosteroids are the first-line therapy. Supplementary treatment is added and the dose of corticosteroids is increased, according to the severity of asthma, in a stepwise fashion (Figure 16). Short-acting β_2 agonists are used as and when needed for episodic bronchoconstriction.

Prophylactic medications

Topical corticosteroids, such as budesonide, are effective anti-inflammatory agents. The onset of effect is slow, over a few days, and the maximum benefit may not be achieved for a few weeks. Adverse effects are mainly local, such as oropharyngeal candidia-

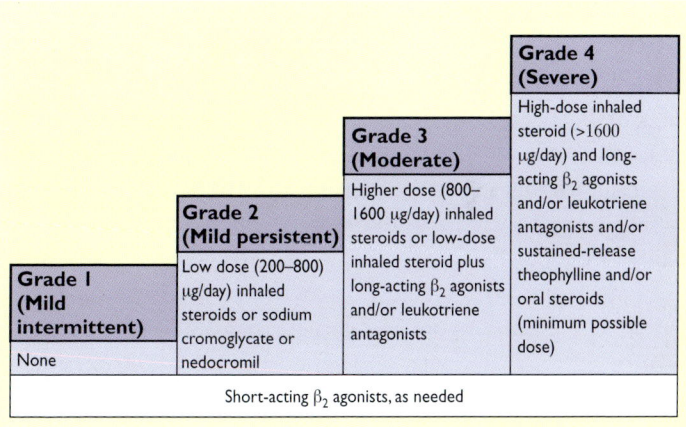

Grade 1 (Mild intermittent)	Grade 2 (Mild persistent)	Grade 3 (Moderate)	Grade 4 (Severe)
None	Low dose (200–800) μg/day) inhaled steroids or sodium cromoglycate or nedocromil	Higher dose (800–1600 μg/day) inhaled steroids or low-dose inhaled steroid plus long-acting β_2 agonists and/or leukotriene antagonists	High-dose inhaled steroid (>1600 μg/day) and long-acting β_2 agonists and/or leukotriene antagonists and/or sustained-release theophylline and/or oral steroids (minimum possible dose)
Short-acting β_2 agonists, as needed			

Figure 16 *Stepwise treatment of asthma. Starting treatment as appropriate to the grade of asthma severity, the level of treatment is moved up if control is not achieved and down once the asthma has been under good control for 3–6 months. Adapted from Global Strategy for Asthma Management and Prevention. NHLBI/WHO Workshop Report. NIH publication 1995; No. 95: 3659.*

sis. Systemic corticosteroids, such as oral prednisolone, are given as short courses for exacerbation, although, in severe asthma, regular medication may be indicated. Side-effects include hypertension, hyperglycaemia, osteoporosis, cataracts, obesity, thinning of skin, muscle weakness and suppression of the hypothalamic–pituitary–adrenal axis.

Sodium cromoglycate and nedocromil sodium are not as potent as steroids, but may be useful where there are concerns about steroid side-effects, such as in children. In the last few years, anti-leukotriene agents have become available. These block the effects of leukotrienes and therefore act as anti-inflammatory agents. These are also less potent than inhaled steroids. The place of anti-leukotriene agents has not been clearly established. They could be used as first-line therapy in mild persistent asthma and/or in patients with moderate-to-severe asthma receiving high-dose inhaled/oral corticosteroids. In severe asthma (steroid dependent/steroid insensitive), immunosuppressive drugs such as methotrexate and cyclosporin could be used. Regular monitoring is required and they should only be used under the supervision of an asthma specialist.

Long-acting bronchodilators include long-acting β_2 agonists such as salmeterol, given as inhaler, and sustained-release theophylline, given as oral therapy. They are useful as regular, adjuvant therapy to inhaled steroids in moderate persistent asthma and are particularly effective for nocturnal symptoms. They should not be used as prophylactic medication on their own. The therapeutic index of theophylline is low, and serious side-effects such as seizures, tachyarrhythmias and central nervous system stimulation can occur with high doses.

Rescue medications

Short acting β_2 agonist (such as salbutamol) are effective bronchodilators used to treat acute symptoms during episodic bronchoconstriction or an exacerbation, mostly through the inhaled route. In high doses, they may cause cardiovascular stimulation, tremor and hypokalaemia. Anticholinergics, such as ipratropium bromide, are less potent than the β_2 agonists, but may have an additive effect.

Allergic rhinoconjunctivitis

The term rhinoconjunctivitis implies inflammation of the nasal and conjunctival mucosa. Therefore, treatment with anti-inflammatory drugs such as steroids and sodium cromoglycate is effective. However, rhinitis is mainly expressed through vascular engorgement, and histamine is the most important mediator. Thus antihistamines are also effective in this disease (Table 2).

Table 2 *Pharmacological treatment of rhinitis.*

Drugs	Frequency	Most effective	Less effective	Important side-effect
First-generation antihistamines (e.g. chlorpheniramine)	Regularly or as required	Sneezing, itching and rhinorrhoea	Nasal blockage	Drowsiness
Second-generation antihistamines (e.g. cetirizine, loratadine)	Regularly or as required	Sneezing, itching and rhinorrhoea	Nasal blockage	Arrhythmias
Topical (nasal) corticosteroids (e.g. beclomethasone)	Regularly, once or twice a day	Nasal blockage and rhinorrhoea	Sneezing and itching	Epistaxis
Topical sodium cromoglycate or nedocromil	Regularly, three to four times a day ·	Nasal blockage and rhinorrhoea	Sneezing and itching	Local irritation
Sympathomimetics (e.g. ephedrine)	3–4 times a day as required	Nasal blockage and rhinorrhoea	Sneezing and itching	Rebound congestion
Anticholinergic (e.g. ipratropium bromide)	3–4 times a day as required	Rhinorrhoea	Nasal blockage, itching, sneezing	Epistaxis

Antihistamines prevent and relieve symptoms such as sneezing, itching, rhinorrhoea and excessive lacrimation, but are less effective in relieving nasal blockage. For chronic symptoms, second-generation antihistamines, such as loratidine or cetirizine, should be given orally, whereas topical (intranasal) antihistamine may be indicated for intermittent symptoms.

Intranasal corticosteroids suppress inflammation and thus reduce nasal congestion and rhinorrhoea. They are effective locally with minimal systemic side-effects, which makes long-term therapy acceptable. Local side-effects include epistaxis. Systemic steroids are sometimes used to treat severe rhinoconjunctivitis not responding adequately to other medications.

Sodium cromoglycate and nedocromil sodium, used topically, are less potent than nasal steroids. They may be used in conjunctivitis and for mild-to-moderate rhinitis, especially in children. Anti-leukotriene agents may be of value in some patients with rhinitis. An anticholinergic drug, ipratropium bromide, used topically in the nose, is effective when watery discharge is a prominent symptom.

Anti-IgE as a therapeutic strategy

6

The available therapeutic strategies to manage allergic diseases consist of attempts either to desensitize the atopic individual to a given allergen or to diminish the ongoing allergic reaction. Anti-IgE as a novel therapeutic alternative was based on the premise that a therapy interfering with the binding of IgE molecules to both high- and low-affinity receptors should reduce the allergen-induced early and late asthmatic responses by preventing the release of mediators from mast cells. In addition, this should decrease the amplification of the inflammatory responses mediated by helper T-cells by preventing IgE-dependent allergen presentation.

Several strategies were conceived and tested to eliminate IgE-derived signal to the mast cells. These include the use of STAT-6 inhibitors, which interfere with the signal transduction of IL-4 and IL-13, IL-4 antagonists and neutralizing antibodies to IL-4 that target IL-4/IL-13 signal for antibody isotype switching and anti-CD23 antibodies. At present, the most promising approach is the neutralization of IgE by antibodies directed against the region of the IgE molecule that interacts with IgE receptors.

Overview of anti-IgE antibody

Much of the work on the development of an anti-IgE preparation for use in humans has relied on animals. More than a decade ago, rabbit-derived polyclonal anti-IgE antibodies given to mice were found to dramatically reduce IgE levels in serum and suppress the number of IgE-producing B-cells. Treatment of mice with a single injection of an anaphylactogenic anti-IgE monoclonal antibody (MAb) during primary immunization reduced serum IgE, but not IgG, to undetectable levels for over 2 months, even when the animals were exposed to antigen on a weekly basis.

With the development of techniques to produce MAb, a non-anaphylactogenic murine MAb that binds to circulating IgE at the same site as the high-affinity receptor has been developed. An important aspect of the development of this compound was that these antibodies do not bind to IgE bound to cells bearing FcεRI or the FcεRII, because the epitope on IgE against which they are directed is already attached to those receptors and is masked. Consequently, the MAb did not attach to cell-bound IgE and the anti-IgE/IgE complex blocked the binding of IgE to its receptors, thereby avoiding mast cell or basophil activation (Figure 17).

These non-anaphylactogenic humanized murine monoclonal antibodies do not interfere with the production of IgM, IgG and IgA by B-cells. They express a high degree of isotype specificity and can therefore selectively neutralize IgE without affecting other antibody classes. With the clear indication that a MAb that is bound to the FcεRI binding region of IgE could influence both immediate and late-phase allergic responses, the stage was set to apply this to the development of a therapy for use in humans.

Designing the anti-IgE antibody

The use of murine anti-human MAb as therapeutic agents was limited by the occurrence of antibody responses after repeated administration of xenogenic antibodies. This antigenic response could decrease the efficacy of these antibodies by reducing their half-lives through the formation of antibody–antiantibody complexes, and can lead to anaphylactic reactions. For this reason, they were humanized. This process involves removing the immunogenic portion of the murine IgG antibody and splicing in its place a corresponding human IgG portion.

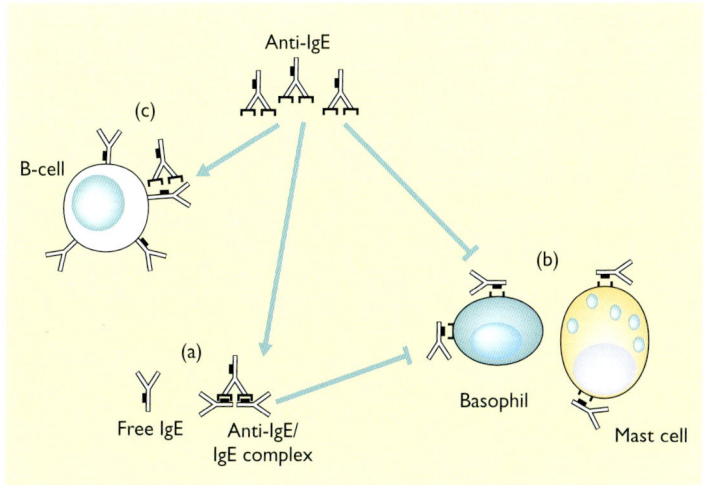

Figure 17 *Mechanism of action of anti-IgE. (a) Anti-IgE binds to free IgE and facilitates its removal. (b) Anti-IgE does not bind to IgE that it is already bound to the IgE receptors on mast cells and basophils. (c) Anti-IgE binds to membrane-bound IgE on B cells inhibiting IgE production by B cells.*

The preparation that meets the ideal requirements for neutralization of IgE antibodies is the recombinant humanized antibody omalizumab (Xolair, rhuMAb-E25). Omalizumab consists of the IgE-binding regions derived from the murine anti-human IgE antibody (MAE11) comprising about 5% of the sequence attached to the human IgG_1 framework that comprises approximately 95% of the sequence, thereby retaining the antigen-binding domain of the murine original. Overall, only three amino acid residues of omalizumab are absent in the human antibody libraries.

Another chimeric MAb (CGP 51901) and a humanized MAb (CGP 56901) were developed from the parent mouse TES-C21. CGP 51901 is a mouse/human chimeric anti-IgE antibody, which consists of the heavy and light chain variable regions of a parent murine antibody and the heavy and light chain constant regions of the human κ and λ1 antibody isotypes. It binds to the low- and high-affinity receptor-binding portions of human IgE located in the Cε3 domain. Chimerization results in reduction of the potential immunogenicity in humans, since 90% of the antibody response is directed against the constant region.

Despite the fact that the two humanized antibodies have similar characteristics, they are directed against separate epitopes on the Cε3 regions of the IgE.

Therapeutic potential

In vitro studies have revealed that the humanized anti-IgE MAb has the following characteristics:

- Binds to free IgE but not to IgA or IgG and reduces the free IgE levels
- Does not bind to mast cell- or basophil-bound IgE
- Blocks the binding of IgE to FcεRI – the high affinity receptors localized on the mast cells, basophils and APCs
- Downregulates the high-affinity receptors on basophils
- Inhibits mast cell degranulation following challenge with rag-weed allergen
- Reduced lung eosinophilia following allergen challenge with decreased production of IL-5 by Th_2 cells.

Pharmacology

Both the chimeric antibody and omalizumab have been tested. In cynamolgous monkeys presensitized with human ragweed-specific IgE, omalizumab injected into the skin reduced the wheal and flare response to ragweed antigen with a 100% response rate after a second dose of omalizumab. Omalizumab also binds to human IgE with equal efficacy. Moreover, omalizumab per se does not stimulate histamine release (Figure 18). Omalizumab has also been shown to decrease levels of both free IgE and FcεRI after each dose in atopic individuals.

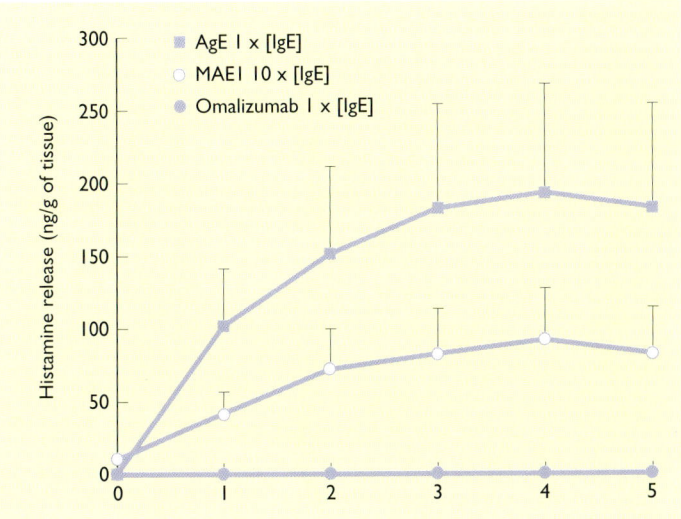

Figure 18 *Omalizumab does not bind to mast cell- or basophil-bound IgE receptors or stimulate histamine release by itself. AgE, antigen E; MAE₁, murine antibody E1. Reproduced with permission of Karger, Basel from Shields et al (1995).*

To achieve therapeutic efficacy with non-anaphylactogenic anti-IgE antibodies, a dose that greatly decreases IgE levels must be used. Since only 2000 IgE molecules are required for a half-maximal release of histamine from basophils exposed to specific allergen, anything less than near complete suppression of IgE levels allows sufficient IgE binding to FcεRI for full basophil activation. This means that anti-IgE dosing needs to be individualized to a patient's total IgE level, and IgE levels during treatment need to be undetectable or nearly so for therapeutic efficacy.

Pharmacokinetics and pharmacodynamics

In preclinical analysis, cynamolgous monkey IgE binds to omalizumab with similar affinity to human IgE ($K_d = 0.19$ nM and 0.06 nM respectively). Omalizumab–IgE complexes have been characterized as small ($<10^6$ Da), and no association has been found with ^{125}I-labelled omalizumab and red cells, indicating that the antibody does not combine with cell-bound IgE. Tissue distribution studies in monkeys did not indicate any specific tissue distribution. The uptake is restricted to the plasma compartment, and omalizumab has a half-life of approximately 5.5 h. Both omalizumab and its complexes are slowly cleared from the blood, and omalizumab–IgE complexes are cleared more rapidly from the circulation than uncomplexed omalizumab. The major route of elimination is through urine, with approximately 50% of the administered dose excreted at 96 h. The serum clearance is greater in animals with higher baseline levels of IgE. Although the elimination of omalizumab–IgE complexes is through the kidneys, the lack of any specific uptake by the kidneys indicates an absence of deposition of these immune complexes in the kidney. The P-K characteristics in children and adolescents have been found to be similar to those in adults after normalization for the weights.

Adverse effects

Animal studies have not shown any evidence of toxicity with administration of up to 100 mg/kg in mice and 50 mg/kg in monkeys, the proposed clinical doses being 2–4 mg/kg. Similarly, multiple doses given three times a week were tolerated well. There were also no reports of anaphylaxis following systemic administration. Furthermore, no significant presence of antibody formation against omalizumab was documented in these studies.

Safety issues

There are at least three safety concerns to be addressed with regard to anti-IgE treatment. These include:

- Causing anaphylaxis
- Predisposing the patient to parasitic infections

- Provoking an immune complex disease through complement fixation or antibody formation

The designing of a non-anaphylactogenic antibody eliminates the apprehension about the development of fatal anaphylaxis.

The second worry relates to the long-held view that IgE is effective in the protection against parasitic infections, and whether blocking of IgE could predispose to parasitic infections. Various studies have yielded mixed results. Amiri and co-workers, after studies on mice treated with rabbit polyclonal anti-mouse IgE, concluded that IgE plays a detrimental rather than a beneficial role for the host in schistosomiasis. Other studies have found that IgE participates in parasite elimination in primary infection with *Schistosoma mansoni* and in the generation of humoral immunity and cytokine response to the parasite. Therefore, the clinical trials on anti-IgE will need to monitor the incidence of parasitic infections in patients treated with anti-IgE.

The third issue regarding anti-IgE treatment was whether anti-IgE could provoke an immune response. The humanization of the antibody and the small size of IgE/anti-IgE complexes are expected to prevent an immune response. It is important to note that the maximal size of immune complexes generated in vitro and in vivo with both CGP 51901 and omalizumab has been two or three IgE molecules with two or three anti-IgE molecules. This size corresponds to that of human IgM, and such complexes are unable to activate complement. A weak antigenic reaction was measured in only one of the subjects treated with the chimeric antibody CGP 51901 and in none of the subjects treated with the humanized omalizumab.

7

Efficacy and safety of anti-IgE in asthma

The possible therapeutic use of anti-IgE in the treatment of patients with asthma was suggested by preliminary proof-of-concept studies in which the antibody demonstrated efficacy in attenuating allergen-induced airway responses. Since antigen challenge represents a good model for mimicking the changes occurring in the airways of subjects with allergic asthma after natural exposure to an allergen, this model has been used in the development of anti-asthmatic drugs to predict the efficacy of newer medications.

Effect of anti-IgE on allergen-induced asthmatic response (phase II trials)

To determine whether omalizumab would be a therapeutic alternative in asthma, studies were conducted to assess its effects on bronchial allergen challenge. The ability of omalizumab to affect the allergen-induced early asthmatic response was tested in a randomized double-blind study. Omalizumab 1 mg/kg produced a significant increase in allergen PC_{15} of 2.2–2.7 doubling doses compared to placebo (−0.8–0.1). The methacholine PC_{20} improved slightly but significantly with omalizumab treatment. The treatment also reduced the total and free unbound IgE levels by 89%, while no changes were observed with placebo.

Another randomized study to investigate the effect of omalizumab on both the early and late asthmatic responses to allergen inhalation showed a significant attenuation of the early asthmatic response, while the magnitude of the late asthmatic response reduced by more than 60% (Figure 19). Furthermore, airway hyper-responsiveness to inhaled methacholine was lower at the end of treatment with omalizumab than before. Treatment with omalizumab also reduced the number of eosinophils in sputum and decreased airway hyper-responsiveness, suggesting that omalizumab has a long-term anti-inflammatory effect.

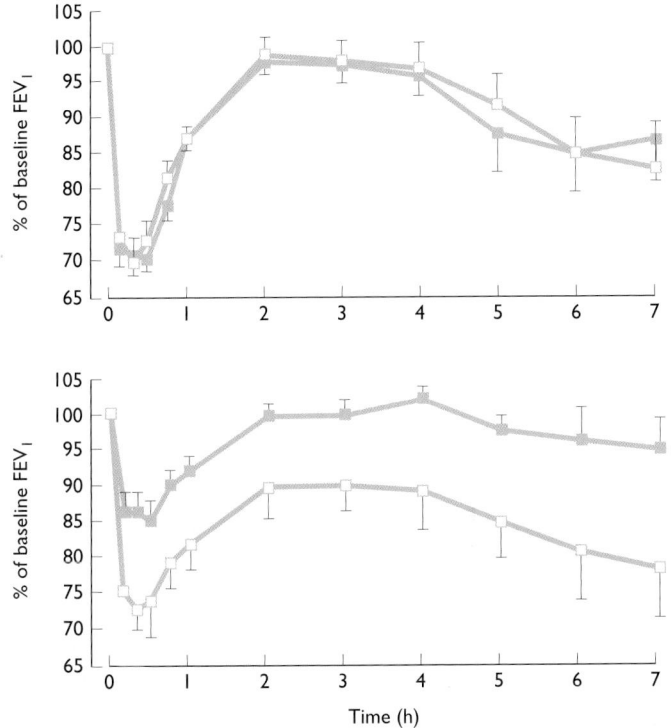

Figure 19 *Effect of omalizumab on allergen-induced early and late asthmatic responses. Changes in FEV$_1$ in the first hour after allergen challenge (early response) and from 2 to 7h after allergen challenge (late response) in placebo (top panel) and omalizumab (lower panel) treated groups are reported as mean percentage of baseline values ± SD before treatment (closed squares). Reproduced with permission from Fahy et al (1997).*

Overall, these studies indicate the therapeutic utility of omalizumab and the first direct evidence of the involvement of IgE in the pathophysiology of the early and late asthmatic responses.

Effect of anti-IgE in allergic asthma (phase III trials)

The phase III programme comprised three large studies in patients with moderate-to-severe allergic asthma receiving conventional treatment with the inhaled corticosteroid beclomethasone dipropionate (BDP) and short-acting β_2-agonists. These included an American study and an international study conducted on 1071 adults and adolescents aged 12–75 years. The third study was conducted in the USA on 334 paediatric patients aged 6–12 years.

The dose of BDP was adjusted during the run-in period to the lowest optimal dose required to maintain control of the asthma symptoms. All studies had a similar design. During the 16 weeks of double-blind treatment, patients were maintained on the baseline dose of BDP without adjustment unless an exacerbation of asthma occurred. In the following 12 weeks, controlled attempts were made to reduce the dose of BDP. Later in the extension phase, the treatment was continued to over a year; this was designed to accumulate data on the safety and tolerability of the medication.

Omalizumab was administered as a subcutaneous injection, and the dose was calculated based on the patients' level of free serum IgE and body weight. The number of exacerbations per patient and the degree of reduction in the dose of BDP were important efficacy variables.

Effect on asthma exacerbations

In the two studies on adults and adolescents, the mean numbers of asthma exacerbations per patient were significantly lower in the omalizumab treatment group during both the study phases. Pooled data showed means of 0.28 and 0.60 exacerbations per patient in the active and placebo groups respectively, during the add-on phase ($p < 0.001$), and 0.38 and 0.71 ($p < 0.001$) during the steroid reduction phase. In the less severe paediatric population, the number of asthma exacerbations was significantly lower with active treatment in the steroid reduction phase alone (0.42 with omalizumab, 0.72 with placebo; $p < 0.001$). During the 1-year treatment period across all three studies, 19 patients required hospital admissions for exacerbations compared with two in the omalizumab group.

Effect on asthma symptom scores and lung function

Likewise, in the two studies on adults and adolescents, significant differences in favour of active treatment were observed for total asthma symptom scores, daily usage of rescue medication and peak expiratory flow rates. These variables remained significantly different in favour of omalizumab during the steroid reduction phase, suggesting that the control of asthma was maintained. Omalizumab treatment resulted in a rapid decrease of serum IgE levels, and this was associated with a concomitant improvement in asthma symptom scores. Improvements in FEV_1 were modest, and active treatment was not significantly different from placebo in this measure.

Steroid-sparing effect

Treatment with omalizumab has resulted in a decreased need for both oral and inhaled corticosteroids (Figure 20). The median percentage reduction in BDP dose achieved was 50% in the placebo treatment groups in the studies in adults and adolescents, compared with 75% and 83% in the active treatment groups of the two studies respectively (both $p < 0.001$). In the paediatric study, patients achieved median BDP reductions of 100% in the omalizumab group and 67% with placebo ($p = 0.001$). Approximately 20% of the placebo-treated patients and 40% of omalizumab-treated patients were able to withdraw from BDP

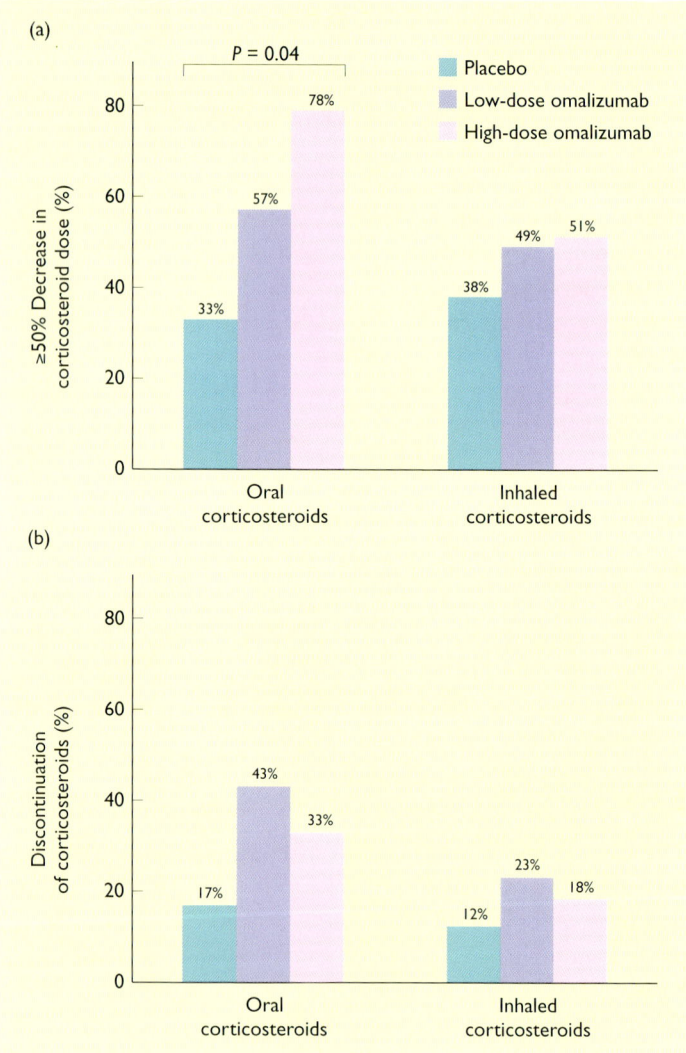

Figure 20 *(a) Percentage of subjects in each group who were able to reduce their daily corticosteroid dose by at least 50% at 20 weeks. (b) Percentage of subjects in each group who were able to discontinue corticosteroid therapy. Reproduced with permission from Milgrom et al (1999). Copyright © 1999 Massachusetts Medical Society. All rights reserved.*

completely in the two adult studies, while the figures in the pae-diatric study were 39% and 55%.

Asthma specific quality of life (AQoL)

Treatment of asthmatic subjects with omulizumab has been shown to improve AQoL scores in both adults and adolescents after 12 weeks and 16 weeks of treatment. Results indicated that improvement in scores were significant over the four areas (activity limitations, asthma symptoms, emotional function and environmental exposure). Clinically meaningful improvements were found to continue even after steroid withdrawal, indicating that omalizumab independently improves AQoL in patients with mild-to-moderate asthma.

Usefulness of anti-IgE in asthma

- Reduces asthma exacerbations
- Improves asthma symptom scores
- Improves lung function
- Improvement in quality of life
- Steroid-sparing effect

Safety and tolerability

The overall profile of adverse events showed little difference between the two treatment groups, and the subcutaneous injec-tion of omalizumab was well tolerated. All the patients in the key phase III studies were tested for anti-omalizumab antibodies at baseline and at follow-up; none developed measurable titres. There was no evidence of immune complex disease or similar syndrome. Treatment appears to be safe and well tolerated in adults, adolescents and paediatric patients with asthma. Systemic urticaria reported from 3.4% of children and 1.4% of adults was the only adverse event considered to have a potential relation-ship to omalizumab administration. The urticaria was mild to moderate in severity and appeared to be highest in children receiving the highest doses. There was no dose relationship in adults. Thus, omalizumab appears safe for human use and can be administered with minimal concern for adverse events.

Efficacy and safety of anti-IgE in allergic rhinitis

8

Allergic rhinitis is a common condition and its prevalence is rising. Although it is not fatal, it causes considerable distress to the sufferer. The cost, in terms of healthcare resources and lost productivity, is considerable. Current therapeutic options – corticosteroids, antihistamines and allergen immunotherapy – provide moderate relief of symptoms, but may be associated with significant adverse effects. Traditional immunotherapy is allergen specific, inconvenient to administer and may occasionally cause serious allergic reactions.

Corticosteroids and antihistamines act at a later stage in the development of allergic inflammation by suppressing the effect of mediators. Allergic rhinitis is closely associated with the presence of specific IgE antibodies to aeroallergens, such as pollen and dust mite. Therefore, blocking the release of IgE-mediated degranulation by humanized monoclonal antibody to IgE (omalizumab) represents a new therapeutic option.

Studies of omalizumab in patients with allergic rhinitis

Perennial allergic rhinitis (house dust mite)

In an open-label study, omalizumab was administered intravenously in 47 patients with perennial allergic rhinitis and a positive skin prick test to dust mites. Depending on their total serum IgE levels, subjects were randomized to receive 0.015 or 0.030 mg/kg per IU per ml of omalizumab every 2 weeks for 182 days. A reduced dosage (0.0015 or 0.005 mg/kg per IU per ml) was administered every two weeks for a further 140 days. Both doses of omalizumab resulted in a ≥ 98% reduction in mean free serum IgE levels compared to baseline and a statistically significant reduction in the mean sums of the wheal areas on skin prick test at day 182 compared to baseline ($p \leq 0.01$). No adverse effects were reported.

Seasonal allergic rhinitis (ragweed)

In a double-blind, placebo-controlled study, 240 subjects were randomized into five groups. The active treatment groups received omalizumab (in mg/kg body weight), 0.15 subcutaneously ($n = 60$) or 0.15 intravenously ($n = 60$) or 0.5 intravenously ($n = 60$) on days 7, 14, 28, 42, 56, 70 and 84. The two remaining groups received placebo, subcutaneously ($n = 20$) or intravenously ($n = 40$). Although serum IgE reduced in a dose-dependent manner, suppression to undetectable levels was observed in only 11 subjects. No significant differences were observed in skin test responses or symptom scores between the groups. The authors concluded that the dose of omalizumab was not adequate to be effective.

Seasonal allergic rhinitis (ragweed)

In another double-blind, placebo-controlled study, 536 subjects were randomized to receive omalizumab 300 mg ($n = 129$), 150 mg ($n = 134$), or 50 mg ($n = 137$), or placebo ($n = 136$). Omalizumab was given subcutaneously every 3 or 4 weeks (depending on the total serum IgE levels), 2 weeks before the start of the pollen season, and continued for 12 weeks. A significant improvement was observed in the occurrence and severity of both nasal and ocular symptoms (Table 3). The requirement for rescue medication was also reduced in the treated group. The investigators demonstrated a dose–response relationship, with the two highest doses providing the greatest relief of symptoms. Apart from urticaria in two patients treated with omalizumab, adverse events were similar in the active treatment and placebo groups. No patients treated with omalizumab developed anti-

Table 3 *Omalizumab in the treatment of ragweed-induced seasonal allergic rhinitis. Subjects receiving the two higher doses had significantly reduced symptom scores and medication requirement.*

	300 mg	150 mg	50 mg	Placebo
DNSS (entire season)	0.75[a]	0.86	0.88	0.98
DNSS (peak pollen season)	0.84[a]	0.95[a]	1.10	1.20
DOSS (entire season)	0.41[a]	0.45[a]	0.49[a]	0.67
Rescue medication (entire season)	0.17[a]	0.20[a]	0.29	0.37

[a]$p < 0.05$.
DNSS, daily nasal symptom score; DOSS, daily ocular symptom score.
Data from Casale et al (1999).

bodies directed against the drug. Further analysis of the data suggests that the efficacy of omalizumab, in terms of improvement in symptoms, is related to its ability to decrease serum free IgE levels. Quality of life, assessed with a standardized questionnaire, was significantly better in patients in the two higher-dose groups (300 mg and 150 mg), compared to placebo.

Seasonal allergic rhinitis (birch pollen)

In a recent double-blind, placebo-controlled study in 251 adult subjects, omalizumab 300 mg or placebo was administered subcutaneously two or three times during the season, depending on the baseline IgE levels. There was a statistically significant improvement in nasal and ocular symptom severity scores, use of antihistamines and quality-of-life scores (Figure 21). Serum free IgE levels decreased markedly in the treated group, and the efficacy was directly related to the extent of reduction in serum IgE. Omalizumab was well tolerated and no anti-omalizumab antibodies were detected.

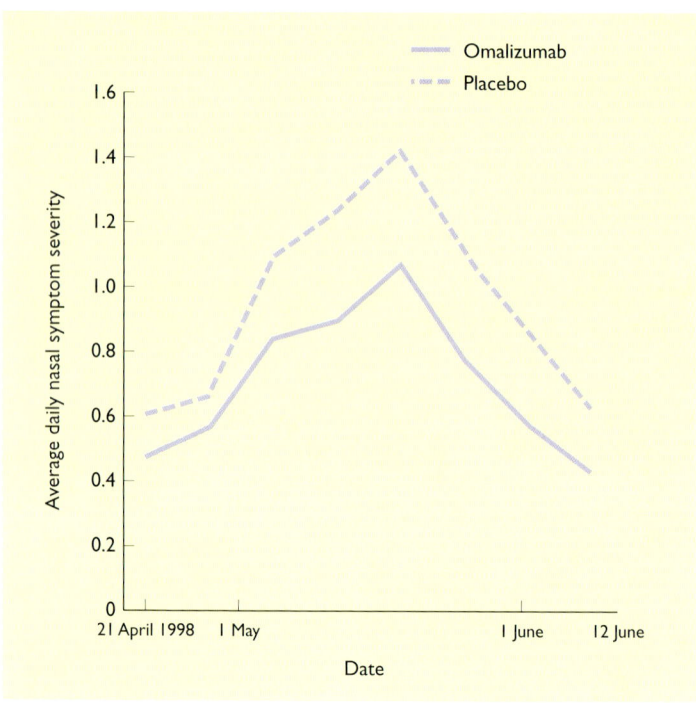

Figure 21 *Omalizumab in the treatment of birch pollen-induced seasonal allergic rhinitis. The average daily nasal symptom severity was considerably reduced in omalizumab treated subjects. Adapted with permission from Adelroth et al (2000).*

Summary of studies

Efficacy

Omalizumab has been shown to be effective in ragweed- and birch pollen-induced seasonal allergic rhinitis. It reduced symptom scores and requirement for rescue medication, and improved quality of life. The improvement is related to the reduction in serum total IgE levels. Its usefulness in perennial allergic rhinitis has recently been investigated.

Safety

Overall, omalizumab is well tolerated. Urticaria has been reported in a few patients. No serious adverse effects have occurred, including anaphylactic or anaphylactoid episodes and complement-related disease. Omalizumab does not stimulate antibody production or formation of immune complexes.

Usefulness of omalizumab in seasonal allergic rhinitis

- Improves nasal and ocular symptom scores
- Reduces rescue medication (antihistamine) requirement
- Improves quality of life

9

Future prospects for IgE in the treatment of allergic disorders

The central role played by IgE in allergic disorders and the ability to lower circulating free IgE with a humanized monoclonal antibody directed against the FcεRI binding domain of IgE represents a novel therapeutic approach for IgE-mediated allergic diseases.

Asthma

In the treatment of asthma, omalizumab has exhibited a prolonged pharmacological effect without inducing anaphylaxis, blunted the early- and late-phase responses to inhaled allergen, reduced the symptoms of asthma and reduced corticosteroid use. However, the optimum duration of treatment with anti-IgE is not clear. The initial findings suggest that patients with asthma where the corticosteroid usage had been reduced with anti-IgE treatment reverted back to their initial status after discontinuation of treatment. However, prolonged suppression of IgE by anti-IgE antibodies will lead to downregulation of the high-affinity FcεRI IgE receptors, thereby inhibiting the IgE-mediated responses in the long run. Omalizumab treatment produces a marked downregulation of FcεRI receptors on basophils from a pretreatment mediator density of about 220 000 receptors per basophil to 8300 receptors per basophil – a decrease of approximately 97%. This, in effect, could further dampen the allergic cascade.

A minority of asthmatics have late-onset asthma associated with negative skin tests to common allergens and normal circulating

IgE. These individuals have non-atopic or 'intrinsic' asthma, which tend to be more severe. These individuals have local sensitization and have been shown to produce IgE widely in their airways, suggesting a role for IgE in these patients. It would be of interest to note whether these individuals would benefit from anti-IgE therapy, either systemically or through the inhalation route.

Immunotherapy

One of the approaches to the treatment and prevention of allergy is desensitization and blockade of effector pathways. In desensitization, the aim is to shift the antibody response away from an IgE-dominated response towards one dominated by IgG, which can prevent the allergen from activating IgE-mediated pathways. Lowering IgE levels with anti-IgE antibodies could be an effective way to undertake allergen-specific immunotherapy. To induce antigen-specific tolerance by allergen-specific immunotherapy, a higher dose of allergen is preferred but this is limited by the appearance of hypersensitivity reactions. For example, peanut allergy, which is severe, is not amenable to allergen immunotherapy due to the high risk of anaphylaxis. Blocking IgE with MAb can be an effective way to initiate allergen immunotherapy.

Anti-IgE could also find a role in the management of patients with co-existent multiple allergies such as food allergies, allergic rhinitis, allergic conjunctivitis and atopic dermatitis. It would be easy to treat the whole gamut of allergies in such an individual with anti-IgE rather than specific medications for relief of each symptom. Furthermore, anti-IgE as a therapeutic alternative could find support in patients suffering from seasonal allergic rhinitis, hay fever and asthma, where anti-IgE therapy during the particular season for 6–8 weeks can abrogate the symptoms. This is also meaningful in the context of adverse effects, considering that there have not been any apparent side-effects detected in the various trials held so far.

Other applications

Treatment of hyper IgE syndrome with anti-IgE antibody is an exciting possibility. However, the high doses of antibody required to neutralize the IgE precludes its use at present.

Another exciting field is the use of anti-IgE antibodies in an acute setting. It would be interesting to note whether anti-IgE could find use in acute anaphylactic reactions and in acute severe asthma. The slow onset of action could preclude its use in an emergency situation.

The possibility of administration of anti-IgE in babies to prevent the development of the allergic march is of interest. As IgE responses are formed in the first 3 years of life, blockade of IgE in at-risk babies could prevent the occurrence of allergic diseases in future.

Safety

An important aspect, which is not yet apparent with the present studies, is the duration of treatment. In case the treatment is to be prolonged over a very long duration to maintain the effects of anti-IgE, the possible chances of adverse effects also loom large. It is generally believed that IgE plays a role in the surveillance and defence against parasitic infections, and whether blocking IgE in the long term will predispose to parasitic infections remains to be seen. Studies done in primates have not shown any conclusive proof that blocking of IgE has increased the prevalence of ascariasis and other nematode infections. There was also no increase in the incidence of threadworm infestation in children who were given anti-IgE for allergic asthma. Though there has been no evidence of adverse effects in the studies conducted so far, the long-term consequences need to be evaluated. This is significant, since the ideal duration of treatment is still not certain.

Anti-IgE therapy is a novel therapeutic alternative in the management of allergic disorders but there are still many unanswered questions regarding this new and exciting molecule. One of the limitations of anti-IgE is that it is a protein that must be given by injection. On the other hand, the subcutaneous route of injection may help improve patient adherence to other recommended management measures through regular visits for treatment. In the future, small molecules with higher affinity for receptors might be developed, but until that time omalizumab represents a significant advance in the development of novel therapies for asthma.

Further reading

Adelroth E, Rak S, Haahtela T et al. Recombinant humanized mAb-E25, an anti-IgE mAb, in birch pollen-induced seasonal allergic rhinitis. *J Allergy Clin Immunol* 2000;**106**(2):253–9.

Barnes PJ. Anti-IgE antibody therapy for asthma. *N Engl J Med* 1999; **341**(26):2006–8.

Barnes PJ. Pathophysiology of allergic inflammation. In: Middleston Jr E, Reed CE, Ellis EF, Adkinson Jr NF, Yuninger JW, Busse WW, eds. *Allergy Principles and Practice,* 5th edn. St Louis, MO: Mosby, 1998: 356–66.

Boulet LP, Chapman KR, Cote J et al. Inhibitory effects of an anti-IgE antibody E25 on allergen-induced early asthmatic response. *Am J Respir Crit Care Med* 1997;**155**(6):1835–40.

Burrows B, Martinez FD, Halonen M et al. Association of asthma with serum IgE levels and skin-test reactivity to allergens. *N Engl J Med* 1989;**320**:271–7.

Busse WW, Horwirz RJ, Reed CE. Asthma, definitions and pathogenesis. In: Middleston Jr E, Reed CE, Ellis EF, Adkinson Jr NF, Yuninger JW, Busse WW, eds. *Allergy Principles and Practice* 5th edn. St Louis, MO: Mosby, 1998:838–58.

Casale TB, Bernstein IL, Busse WW et al. Use of an anti-IgE humanized monoclonal antibody in ragweed-induced allergic rhinitis. *J Allergy Clin Immunol* 1997;**100**:110-21.

Casale T, Condemi J, Miller SD et al. rhuMAb-E25 in the treatment of seasonal allergic rhinitis (SAR). *Ann Allergy Asthma Immunol* 1999;**82**:75.

Corne J, Djukanovic R, Thomas L et al. The effect of intravenous administration of a chimeric anti-IgE antibody on serum IgE levels in atopic subjects: efficacy, safety, and pharmacokinetics. *J Clin Invest* 1997;**99**(5):879–87.

Corry DB, Kheradmand F. Induction and regulation of the IgE response. *Nature* 1999;**402**:B18–23.

Fahy JV, Cockcroft DW, Boulet LP et al. Effect of aerosolized anti-IgE (E25) on airway responses to inhaled allergen in asthmatic subjects. *Am J Respir Crit Care Med* 1999;**160**(3):1023–7.

Fahy JV, Fleming HE, Wong HH, Liu JT et al. The effect of an anti-IgE monoclonal antibody on the early-and-late phase responses to allergen inhalation in asthmatic subjects. *Am J Respir Crit Care Med* 1997;**155**:1828–34.

Global strategy for asthma management and prevention. NHLBI/WHO Workshop Report. NIH publication No. 95-3659. Bethesda, MD: National Institutes of Health, 1995.

Holgate ST. The cellular and mediator basis of asthma in relation to natural history. *Lancet* 1997;**350** (Suppl 2):SII5–9.

Holgate ST. The epidemic of allergy and asthma. *Nature* 1999; **402** (suppl):B2–4.

Holgate ST, Corne J, Jardieu P et al. Treatment of allergic airways disease with anti-IgE. *Allergy* 1998;**53**:83–8.

Holt PG, Macaubas C, Stumbles PA, Sly PD. The role of allergy in the development of asthma. *Nature* 1999;**402** (suppl):B12–17.

Milgrom H, Fick RBJ, Su JQ et al. Treatment of allergic asthma with monoclonal anti-IgE antibody. rhuMAb-E25 Study Group. *N Engl J Med* 1999;**341**(26):1966–73.

Mygind N, Dahl R, Pedersen S, Thestrup-Pedersen K. Essential allergy. In: *Rhinitis*, 2nd edn. Oxford: Blackwell Science Ltd, 1996:195–252.

National Institute of Health, National Heart, Lung, and Blood Institute. *Highlights of the Expert Panel Report II: Guidelines for the Diagnosis and Management of Asthma*, NIH Publication 97-4051A. Bethesda, Md: NIH, 1997.

Nelson HS. Asthma guidelines and outcomes. In: Middleston Jr E, Reed CE, Ellis EF, Adkinson Jr NF, Yuninger JW, Busse WW, eds. *Allergy Principles and Practice,* 5th edn. St Louis, MO: Mosby, 1998:927–37.

Oddera S, Silvestri M, Penna R et al. Airway eosinophilic inflammation and bronchial hyperresponsiveness after allergen inhalation challenge in asthma. *Lung* 1998;**176**(4):237–47.

Oettgen HC, Geha RS. IgE in asthma and atopy: cellular and molecular connections. *J Clin Invest* 1999;**104**(7):829–35.

Patalano F. Injection of anti-IgE antibodies will suppress IgE and allergic symptoms. *Allergy* 1999;**54**(2):103–10.

Shields RL, Whether WR, Zioncheck K et al. Inhibition of allergic reactions with antibodies to IgE. *Int Arch Allergy Immunol* 1995; **107**(1–3):308–12.

Tariq SM, Matthews SM, Hakim EA et al. The prevalence of and risk factors for atopy in early childhood: A birth cohort study. *J Allergy Clin Immunol* 1998;**101**:587–93.

Index